ILEOANAL POUCH SURGERY NUTRITION

Complete Guide Unlocking The Secrets Of
Nutrition To Rapid Healing After Surgery
Success, Nourishing Meal Plans, Recipes, Tips
For Optimal Health Wellness)

DR. ALLAN FREDA

Contents

1. Description of the Procedure: Detailed descriptions of the advantages and possible drawbacks of ileoanal pouch surgery.

2. Nutrition Essentials: Comprehensive details on what people should eat after surgery, emphasizing the role that vitamins, minerals, and macronutrients have in the healing process.

3. Recipes for Healing: A selection of dishes created specially to promote digestive health and assist in recuperation. Nutrient-dense, easily digested foods are the main emphasis of these dishes.

4. Meal Plans: Personalised meal plans to assist people in efficiently organizing their food following surgery. These meal plans ensure sufficient nutrients for healing while accommodating dietary preferences and limits.

5. Expert Advice: Guidance from medical specialists and dietitians on addressing nutritional difficulties following surgery, handling possible side effects, and preserving long-term health.

All things considered, this book provides an extensive manual for navigating the dietary elements of recovering from ileoanal pouch surgery. Giving readers the information and tools, they need to optimize their diet for healing and long-term health, empowers them.

OVERVIEW

Patients with ulcerative colitis or familial adenomatous polyposis (FAP) are the main candidates for ileoanal pouch surgery, commonly referred to as ileal pouch-anal anastomosis (IPAA) or J-pouch surgery. By removing the colon and rectum and creating a pouch from the small intestine that is attached to the anus, this surgical procedure enables waste to be eliminated without the need for a long-term ostomy. By addressing symptoms like diarrhea, bleeding in the rectal area, and abdominal pain, the procedure seeks to enhance the patient's quality of life. It is typically taken into consideration in cases of problems such as dysplasia linked with colitis or cancer, or when all other medical therapy options have been tried.

Nutrition's Function in the Healing Process After Surgery:

For patients undergoing ileoanal pouch surgery, nutrition is essential to the healing process following surgery. A balanced diet can promote general health and wellness, lower the risk of problems, and speed up the healing of wounds. Patients may have changes in digestion, absorption, and bowel function after surgery; therefore, dietary adjustments are necessary to maximize nutrient intake and foster healing. Furthermore, pouchitis—a common complication marked by inflammation of the pouch—can be influenced by specific dietary components, underscoring the need for nutrition in post-surgery treatment.

This extensive guide will go over the dietary suggestions and considerations for patients having ileoanal pouch surgery. It includes recovery recipes, meal plans, and professional advice for long-term health.

Dietary Guidelines for Recuperation Following Surgery:

1. Moving to a Low-Residue Diet: To reduce intestinal discomfort and encourage recovery, patients who have had ileoanal pouch surgery are frequently encouraged to move to a low-residue diet. Consuming high-fiber foods like whole grains, unprocessed fruits and vegetables, nuts, and seeds is restricted in a low-residue diet since they can be difficult to digest and aggravate symptoms like diarrhea and upset stomach. To supply vital nutrients without taxing the digestive system, the focus is instead on ingesting meals

that are simple to digest, such as prepared fruits and vegetables, lean meats, refined grains, and well-cooked cereals.

2. Tracking Fibre Intake: Although a low-residue diet is advised at first, reinstating foods high in fiber gradually will improve overall gastrointestinal health and colon function. But it's crucial to keep an eye on your intake of fiber and pick well-tolerated sources, such as cooked veggies, soft fruits, and soluble fiber supplements like psyllium husk. Particularly in the early stages of recovery, insoluble fiber—found in foods like bran and raw vegetables—should be taken in moderation as it might aggravate the colon and increase the frequency of stools.

3. Stressing Foods High in Protein: Protein is a necessary nutrient for recovering after surgery since it aids in tissue repair and wound healing. Consuming foods high in protein, such as fish, chicken, eggs, lentils, tofu, and lean meats, can aid

in the body's healing processes and aid in the rebuilding of muscle tissue. Furthermore, protein aids in satiety promotion and blood sugar stabilization, both of which are particularly helpful for people who are experiencing changes in appetite and energy levels after surgery.

4. Maintaining Appropriate Hydration: Staying properly hydrated is critical for preserving regular bowel movements, avoiding dehydration, and promoting general health and well-being.

After ileoanal pouch surgery, patients may lose more fluids due to sweating, diarrhea, and wound drainage; therefore, staying properly hydrated is essential to avoiding electrolyte imbalances and dehydration. To assist replace lost fluids and encourage hydration, drink lots of water throughout the day and eat meals high in water content, such as fruits, vegetables, and soups.

5. Controlling Fat Intake: Although fat is a necessary component that gives us energy and aids

in the absorption of other nutrients, some fats might make symptoms worse for people who already have digestive problems, such as diarrhea and stomach pain.

Reduce your intake of high-fat foods after surgery, especially those that are fried, oily, or highly processed, as these can be difficult to digest and may cause gastrointestinal distress. Instead, concentrate on introducing moderation in the consumption of healthier fats such as those found in nuts, seeds, avocados, olive oil, and avocados to promote general health and wellness.

Ideas for Meal Planning and Recipes:

1. Breakfast: Begin the day with a filling and simple-to-digest meal, like scrambled eggs with spinach and feta cheese or muesli topped with sliced bananas and a drizzle of honey. Alternatively, for a vitamin and mineral boost, whip up a delicious smoothie with Greek yogurt, mixed berries, and a handful of spinach.

2. Lunch: Have a quinoa salad with grilled chicken, mixed veggies, and a lemon vinaigrette dressing for a filling and healthy midday meal. Alternatively, use low-residue items like potatoes, zucchini, and carrots to make a pot of flavorful vegetable soup that is seasoned with herbs and spices.

3. Dinner should be light and savory, such as roasted chicken with mashed sweet potatoes and sautéed green beans, or grilled salmon with steamed broccoli and quinoa pilaf. Try varying the herbs, spices, and marinades you use to improve the flavor of your food without sacrificing nutritional value.

4. Snacks: Stock up on healthy snacks like hummus with carrot sticks and cucumber slices, Greek yogurt with honey and almonds, or sliced apples with peanut butter in case you get hungry in between meals. These snacks provide you with

the right balance of fiber, healthy fats, and protein to keep you full and focused all day.

Professional Advice for Long-Term Health:

1. Consult a trained Dietitian: Throughout the post-surgery recuperation period and beyond, a trained dietitian can offer individualized nutritional counsel and assistance. A dietitian may assist in developing a personalized meal plan based on your specific requirements, address any dietary limitations or worries, and provide helpful advice on how to maximize nutrient intake and support long-term wellness.

2. Maintain a Food Diary: Measuring your food intake and symptoms in a food diary can assist in identifying foods or patterns that may act as triggers for gastrointestinal symptoms including bloating, diarrhea, or abdominal pain.

You may make more educated decisions to promote your general well-being and gain a better understanding of how different foods affect your digestive health by keeping a journal of your meals, snacks, and symptoms.

3. Engage in Mindful Eating: This type of eating entails focusing on the flavors, textures, and aromas of the meal as well as your body's signals of hunger and fullness.

You may improve digestion, lessen overeating, and strengthen your bond with food by engaging in mindful eating practices including chewing carefully, appreciating each bite, and paying attention to your body's signals of hunger and fullness.

4. Remain Active: Maintaining general health and well-being, especially for those recuperating from surgery, requires regular physical activity. Try to fit in regular exercise to your daily schedule, such as yoga, weight training, swimming, or walking, to help with digestion, circulation, and muscle strength. Before beginning any new fitness program, make sure to speak with your healthcare

professional, especially if you have any medical ailments or concerns.

for patients having ileoanal pouch surgery, nutrition is critical to the healing process following surgery. Patients can maximize healing, lower the risk of problems, and foster long-term well-being by adhering to a well-balanced diet that prioritizes nutrient-rich foods, minimizes irritants, and supports gastrointestinal health. After surgery, incorporating meal plans, healing recipes, and professional advice into your daily routine can support your journey back to optimal health and energy. Always seek the advice of your trained dietician and medical team for customized guidance and assistance during your recuperation.

CHAPTER 1
GETTING READY FOR SURGERY

Patients must prepare physically and psychologically before having ileoanal pouch surgery, with special attention to their dietary health. Dietary recommendations made before surgery are essential for achieving the best possible results for both the operation and the healing phase that follows. These recommendations usually combine dietary considerations with meal planning and preparation techniques catered to the individual's requirements.

Pre-operative food Guidelines: To maximize their nutritional status and get their bodies ready for ileoanal pouch surgery, patients are frequently encouraged to adhere to particular food guidelines before the procedure. Depending on the patient's general health, underlying medical issues, and the particular needs of the surgical team, these recommendations may change. However, standard advice frequently consists of:

1. High Protein Intake: Patients undergoing surgery must consume enough protein because it is necessary for tissue regeneration and wound healing. Adequate protein consumption helps enhance immune system function, encourage healing, and sustain muscular mass. Lean meats, poultry, fish, eggs, dairy products, legumes, nuts, and seeds are among the food's high in protein.

2. Sufficient Hydration: To promote general health and enhance recuperation, it's imperative to keep the right amount of water before surgery. Dehydration raises the possibility of complications and hinders the healing of wounds. Patients are usually recommended to limit their intake of coffee and alcohol and to drink lots of fluids, such as water, herbal teas, and electrolyte-rich drinks.

3. Diet: A balanced diet rich in a range of nutrient-dense meals is crucial to getting the body ready for surgery. To supply vital vitamins, minerals, antioxidants, and fiber, this entails consuming an abundance of fruits, vegetables, whole grains, and healthy fats. Reducing intake of processed foods, sugary snacks, and high-fat foods can improve general health and nutritional status.

4. Vitamin and Mineral Supplementation: To treat specific nutritional deficiencies or promote optimal recovery, patients may occasionally need additional vitamin and mineral supplementation.

Zinc, vitamin D, calcium, iron, and vitamin B12 are examples of common supplements. To guarantee safety and effectiveness, it is imperative to speak with a healthcare provider before beginning any new supplement regimen.

Before Surgery: To promote the best possible results and lower the risk of problems, patients having ileoanal pouch surgery should take into account several nutritional considerations in addition to adhering to pre-operative dietary guidelines.

These factors could consist of:

1. Resolving Nutritional Deficiencies: Before surgery, patients who suffer from underlying nutritional deficiencies, such as iron deficiency anemia or vitamin inadequacies, may find it helpful to take certain supplements or follow dietary recommendations. Improving overall health outcomes and nutritional status can be achieved by addressing these deficiencies.

2. Managing Inflammatory Bowel Disease (IBD): It's critical to control symptoms and minimize inflammation before surgery for individuals with underlying IBD, such as Crohn's disease or ulcerative colitis. This could entail adhering to a particular diet, like a low-residue or low-fermentable-carbohydrate diet (FODMAPs) diet,

to reduce gastrointestinal symptoms and maximize healing.

3. Avoiding Trigger items: People who suffer from IBD or other gastrointestinal disorders should steer clear of items like dairy, coffee, spicy cuisine, and high-fiber foods that might aggravate their symptoms. Before surgery, identifying and avoiding trigger foods might help reduce gastrointestinal discomfort and accelerate healing.

4. Pre-operative counseling: Patients can receive individualized nutritional advice and support by scheduling a consultation with a trained dietitian or nutritionist before surgery. During the pre-operative phase, these experts can assist in addressing particular nutritional issues, creating customized meal plans, and offering useful tips for meal preparation and administration.

Meal Planning and Preparation: Ensuring that patients have access to wholesome meals that promote healing and rehabilitation is a crucial part of getting ready for ileoanal pouch surgery.

Before surgery, patients should think about the following while making food plans:

1. Nutrient Density: To promote healing and recuperation, emphasize including nutrient-dense foods that offer vital vitamins, minerals, and antioxidants. To maximize dietary intake, prioritize whole grains, fruits, vegetables, lean meats, and healthy fats in meals and snacks.

2. Portion Control: Be mindful of serving sizes and strive to eat well-balanced meals that satisfy your need for calories and nutrients without going overboard. Before and after surgery, portion restriction can help avoid pain, bloating, and digestive problems.

3. Meal Frequency: For people with gastrointestinal disorders, eating smaller, more frequent meals throughout the day might help manage symptoms and improve digestion. To

sustain energy levels and enhance overall nutritional intake, try to eat every three to four hours.

4. Meal Preparation Techniques: To reduce gastrointestinal pain, use culinary techniques like steaming, boiling, baking, or grilling that are easy on the digestive system. Steer clear of highly processed or fried foods, as they can be difficult to digest and worsen symptoms.

Patients can optimize their nutritional status and support optimal outcomes for ileoanal pouch surgery by adhering to pre-operative dietary guidelines, thinking through nutritional factors before surgery, and putting into practice efficient meal planning and preparation procedures.

To ensure that patients are well-prepared for surgery and the ensuing recovery process, close collaboration with healthcare specialists, such as certified dietitians and nutritionists, may offer crucial support and direction during the pre-operative period.

CHAPTER 2
NUTRITION FOR POST-SURGERY RECOVERY

An adequate diet is crucial for achieving the best possible recovery and long-term health after ileoanal pouch surgery. This extensive manual explores all the important topics related to nutrition after surgery, including how to proceed with the first diet, how to handle stomach adjustments, and how to include the necessary nutrients. It is crucial for people navigating the healing process following ileoanal pouch surgery to comprehend these ideas.

First Dietary Advancement Following Surgery

Significant physiological changes occur in the post-ileoanal pouch surgical period, and dietary alterations are crucial to promote healing and reduce discomfort.

Patients usually start with a clear liquid diet to give their digestive tracts time to heal and rest.

Clear liquids that are easy to digest, such as juice, broth, and gelatin, minimize digestive strain while providing hydration and readily absorbed nutrients. As tolerance increases, the diet moves towards refined carbohydrates, lean protein sources, and low-fiber, readily digested meals such as prepared fruits and vegetables. It is important to gradually increase the diet while keeping an eye out for any indications of discomfort or intolerance.

The diet can progressively include more complex carbs, foods high in fiber, and healthy fats as the gastrointestinal tract heals. These nutrient-dense foods boost overall nutritional status, encourage satiety, and offer sustained energy. But it's crucial to introduce these meals gradually and keep an eye out for any negative side effects, such as gas, bloating, or diarrhea. Ensuring appropriate nutrient intake during the recovery process and customizing the diet to individual needs can be achieved by collaborating closely with a qualified dietitian or healthcare professional.

Handling Digestionary Shifts

Significant changes to digestive function, such as altered bowel habits and absorption capacities, are frequently the consequence of ileoanal pouch surgery. Patients may have more frequent bowel movements, notice changes in the consistency of their feces, and find it difficult to tolerate specific foods. It is crucial to adopt dietary practices that support gastrointestinal health and minimize symptoms to effectively manage these digestive alterations.

Keeping enough water in mind is essential for regulating changes in the digestive system. Sustaining digestive function, avoiding dehydration, and enhancing general well-being all depend on maintaining optimal hydration levels. Drinking lots of fluids—such as electrolyte-rich beverages, herbal teas, and water—can support healthy bowel movements and help ward off constipation. Limiting the consumption of drying substances like alcohol and caffeine can also help with hydration efforts.

Post-surgery digestive health can also be supported by incorporating fermentable fibers, like those found in fruits, vegetables, legumes, and whole grains. By acting as prebiotics, these fibers support a healthy microbiome and feed beneficial gut flora. However, since some people may be sensitive to specific kinds of fermentable carbs, it is crucial to introduce these fibers gradually and watch for any negative reactions.

Additionally, controlling meal frequency and portion amounts might help reduce discomfort and bloating associated with digestive issues.

Smaller, more frequent meals spread out throughout the day can help improve food tolerance and ease the burden on the digestive system.

Eating slowly and fully chewing food can also improve digestion and reduce the chance of gastrointestinal upset.

Including Crucial Nutrients

After ileoanal pouch surgery, optimal nutrition is crucial for promoting healing and recuperation. Including a wide range of vital nutrients in the diet helps enhance general health and well-being, lessen inflammation, and encourage tissue repair. Omega-3 fatty acids, protein, vitamins, and minerals are important nutrients to pay attention to.

Protein is especially crucial for wound healing and tissue repair after surgery. Lean meats, chicken, fish, eggs, dairy products, lentils, and tofu are examples of high-quality protein sources that can be included in the diet to aid in the body's healing process. To help fulfill increasing protein needs throughout the day, include protein-rich snacks such as Greek yogurt, almonds, and seeds.

Minerals and vitamins are vital for general health and well-being and are involved in many physiological processes. Eating a wide variety of fruits, vegetables, healthy grains, and lean meats will help guarantee that the body gets enough of the important vitamins and minerals.

Nonetheless, certain people might need supplements to help with particular vitamin deficits or to aid in the healing process after surgery.

To determine any dietary deficiencies and create a customized supplementing plan when necessary, working with a healthcare professional or registered dietitian can be beneficial.

Omega-3 fatty acids have anti-inflammatory qualities and can help lessen inflammation and accelerate healing after surgery. They can be found in fatty fish, flaxseeds, chia seeds, walnuts, and algae. Regular consumption of these foods can assist the body's natural healing processes and advance general health and well-being.

after ileoanal pouch surgery, an adequate diet is critical for fostering long-term well-being and supporting recovery. People can effectively manage digestive changes, minimize discomfort, and attain optimal health results by adhering to a progressive diet progression and including important nutrients in their diet. Dietary suggestions can be specifically tailored to each person's needs by collaborating closely with trained dietitians and healthcare specialists, which can assist ensure a successful recovery process.

CHAPTER 3
DEVELOPING A BALANCED DIET

For those having ileoanal pouch surgery, eating a balanced diet is essential because it can have a big impact on their recovery and long-term health results. The foundation of post-surgery nutrition is preparing nutrient-rich meals that give the body the vital nutrients it needs to recover, restore strength, and preserve general wellness. Patients can optimize their nutrient intake and aid in the healing process by emphasizing a wide variety of foods.

Preparing Meals High in Nutrients:

Creating nutrient-dense meals means combining items from every food group to guarantee a sufficient intake of vital elements. The aim is to emphasise whole foods with minimal processing, like fruits, vegetables, whole grains, lean meats, and healthy fats.

These foods are a great source of the vitamins, minerals, antioxidants, and phytonutrients needed to support general health and aid in healing.

A broad intake of vitamins, minerals, and fiber can be ensured by including a colorful array of fruits and vegetables in meals, in addition to adding flavor and variety. Whole grains offer more fiber to support digestive health and complex carbs for long-lasting energy, like quinoa, brown rice, oats, and whole wheat. Lean protein sources such as fish, chicken, tofu, lentils, and eggs are essential for the regeneration of muscles and the repair of damaged tissue after surgery.

The Role of Protein in Recuperation

After ileoanal pouch surgery, protein is essential to the healing process. It is necessary for muscle regeneration, wound healing, and tissue repair. Consuming enough protein speeds up healing and lowers the chance of problems by strengthening and rebuilding tissues that may have been harmed during surgery.

Patients may be able to fulfill their higher protein requirements throughout the recovery phase by including meals high in protein at every meal and snack. Lean protein sources: Fish, poultry, eggs, tofu, lentils, and poultry are good options because they are high-quality sources of protein without having a lot of added sugars or saturated fat. Smoothies or protein drinks can also be easy choices for people who might have trouble eating solid foods just after surgery.

Maximising Intake of Micronutrients:

Optimizing the consumption of micronutrients is essential for maintaining general health and well-being after surgery, in addition to macronutrients such as protein, carbs, and fats. Micronutrients, such as vitamins and minerals, are necessary for several physiological functions, such as wound healing, bone health, and immunological function.

The best approach to guarantee a sufficient intake of micronutrients is to include a wide variety of nutrient-dense foods. Vitamins, minerals, and antioxidants abound in fruits and vegetables, and each color of the fruit or vegetable signifies a distinct phytonutrient with its own set of health advantages. Citrus fruits are a great source of vitamin C, which is necessary for collagen formation and immune system function, while leafy greens like spinach and kale are high in vitamin K, which is important for blood clotting and bone health.

Nuts, seeds, legumes, and whole grains are also excellent providers of minerals like zinc, magnesium, and B vitamins. A varied intake of these items can help avoid dietary deficits and encourage the best possible healing and recuperation after surgery.

A Complete Guide To The Best Post-Surgery Diet, With Healing Recipes, Meal Plans, And Professional Advice For Long-Term Wellness:

It can be difficult to navigate the post-surgery phase, particularly in terms of diet and nutrition.

A thorough guide to the ideal post-surgery diet gives people the information and tools they need to make wise food decisions, encourage healing, and maintain long-term health. This cookbook, meal plans, and professional advice are all included in this handbook, which is specifically designed for people recovering from ileoanal pouch surgery.

Nutrient-rich foods with well-established therapeutic benefits are included in healing recipes to promote and nourish the healing process. These dishes frequently highlight whole, minimally processed foods that are soft on the stomach and easy to digest. Soft-textured foods, smoothies, stews, and soups are popular options since they can be easier to tolerate, particularly in the early post-surgery phase.

Meal plans provide organized instructions on how to split up meals and snacks throughout the day to guarantee sufficient nutrient intake and encourage the best possible recuperation.

A thoughtfully created meal plan provides a road map for a balanced diet throughout the recuperation process by taking into consideration each person's unique dietary preferences, food tolerances, and nutritional requirements. A range of nutrient-dense meals from all food groups may be included in meal plans, with an emphasis on foods high in protein, fruits, vegetables, whole grains, and healthy fats.

Expert advice on navigating the post-surgery diet can be found in the advice of healthcare specialists, such as nutritionists or registered dietitians.

These pointers could be for preventing vitamin shortages, treating particular symptoms or dietary restrictions, or keeping a balanced diet for long-term health and well-being. People can effectively assist their recovery journey and optimize their nutrition by implementing professional recommendations into their everyday routine.

developing a balanced diet, emphasising nutrient-dense meals, placing a high value on protein consumption, and maximizing micronutrient intake are crucial elements of post-surgical nutrition for patients having ileoanal pouch surgery. A thorough guide to the ideal post-surgery diet that includes therapeutic recipes, meal plans, and professional advice can be of immeasurable assistance and direction to people as they navigate the healing process and strive for long-term health.

CHAPTER 4
MANAGING DIGESTIVE SYMPTOMS

After ileoanal pouch surgery, patients' quality of life may be greatly impacted by digestive issues. Although this surgical technique can provide relief from illnesses like familial adenomatous polyposis or ulcerative colitis, it can also present new issues about nutrition and digestion. It is essential to know how to successfully manage these symptoms to guarantee the best possible health and well-being following surgery.

Handling Pain in the Digestive System

Abdominal pain, cramps, and bloating are among the digestive discomforts that people may feel after ileoanal pouch surgery. Changes in bowel function and the digestive system's response to the altered anatomical shape are the likely causes of these symptoms.

An interdisciplinary strategy that includes dietary adjustments, lifestyle alterations, and, in certain situations, medical interventions is necessary to address intestinal discomfort.

Concentrating on ingesting easily digested meals is one dietary approach to reduce stomach discomfort. These consist of low-fiber carbohydrates, lean meats, and cooked vegetables since they are less likely to upset the digestive tract. A healthy balance of gut flora can also be promoted by including probiotic-rich foods like yogurt and fermented veggies, which may help lessen the symptoms of gas and bloating. Foods that are known to cause digestive problems, like fatty, spicy, and artificially sweetened foods, must be avoided since they may worsen symptoms.

Eating smaller, more frequent meals throughout the day is a crucial part of reducing stomach discomfort.

This strategy can lessen the likelihood of cramps and bloating by avoiding overtaxing the digestive system.

Drinking lots of water to stay hydrated is also crucial for preserving digestive health and avoiding constipation, which can exacerbate discomfort in the abdomen.

When treating certain digestive ailments, people may find that taking over-the-counter or prescription drugs helps. Anti-gas drugs can lessen bloating and flatulence, while anti-spasmodic drugs can aid with stomach cramps. Before beginning any new pharmaceutical regimen, it is imperative to speak with a healthcare provider, as they can offer tailored advice based on each patient's unique needs and medical background.

All things considered, managing gastrointestinal distress following ileoanal pouch surgery necessitates a multifaceted strategy that includes dietary changes, lifestyle adjustments, and if required, medicinal interventions.

As they adjust to the changes in their digestive systems, people can reduce discomfort and enhance their general quality of life by putting these ideas into practice.

Dietary Techniques for Bloating and Gas

Bloating and gas are typical digestive symptoms that people who have had ileoanal pouch surgery encounter. Even though these symptoms can be upsetting and painful, there are nutritional approaches that can help reduce them and support comfortable digestion.

Avoiding foods that are known to induce gas and bloating is one dietary tactic to lessen these symptoms. Among them are foods that cause gas, such as broccoli, cabbage, onions, lentils, beans, and carbonated drinks. Reduced consumption of certain items can help people feel less likely to bloat and have a lot of gas.

Increasing the amount of fiber in the diet gradually is another beneficial dietary strategy. Although fiber is necessary for healthy digestion, consuming too much of it too soon can make bloating and gas symptoms worse, especially in people with sensitive digestive systems. Rather, it is best to increase fiber consumption gradually over time, beginning with soluble fiber supplements and easily digestible sources of fiber such as cooked vegetables.

Efficient chewing of meals can also lessen bloating and gas. Food that has been thoroughly chewed breaks down into smaller particles that are easier to digest and less likely to ferment in the gut, which can result in the generation of gas. Eating slowly and deliberately can also help with digestion and reduce the likelihood of swallowing too much air, which can cause bloating.

By including foods high in probiotics in the diet, one can support a balanced population of gut bacteria and potentially alleviate bloating and gas symptoms.

Probiotics from foods like yogurt, kefir, sauerkraut, and kimchi are good for your digestive system and can help ease discomfort. Furthermore, certain people may benefit from taking probiotic supplements, particularly those who have experienced prolonged antibiotic therapy or who have gut microbiota imbalances.

Managing Frequent Bowel Movements

Another typical problem for those who have had ileoanal pouch surgery is bowel frequency.

Even though the increased frequency of bowel movements is a typical adaptation process, it can still be difficult to control, especially in the early stages of recovery. A mix of dietary changes, lifestyle adjustments, and supporting techniques to support bowel health and regularity are needed to cope with constipation.

Focusing on eating foods that are easy on the digestive system and less likely to irritate or produce urgency is one dietary technique to manage bowel frequency. These consist of cooked vegetables, lean proteins, and low-fiber carbs such as white rice, pasta, and bread. Keeping away from items that are known to make bowel frequency worse, like alcohol, coffee, and spicy foods, can also aid with symptom management.

Including soluble fiber in the diet helps support regularity and assists control of bowel motions. In the digestive tract, soluble fiber absorbs water to create a gel-like substance that softens stools and slows down transit, which lowers the frequency of bowel movements. Soluble fiber can be found in psyllium husk, flaxseeds, barley, and oats.

To avoid constipation and preserve gut health, it's critical to progressively increase fiber consumption and drink lots of water.

Keeping a regular eating schedule might also aid in controlling the frequency of bowel movements.

The digestive tract of the body can be trained to anticipate food intake and encourage more regular bowel movements by eating meals at regular times every day. Furthermore, avoiding heavy snacks and large meals right before bed will assist decrease bowel urgency and disturbances at night.

Deep breathing exercises, yoga, and meditation are examples of stress-reduction practices that can be incorporated to assist manage stress and worry, which can worsen bowel frequency.

It has been demonstrated that stress alters the motility and function of the gut, resulting in more frequent bowel movements and gastrointestinal pain. People can improve their overall digestive health and lessen the symptoms of bowel frequency by including relaxation techniques in their everyday activities.

Sometimes people can control their bowel frequency with the use of dietary supplements or medicines. Bulking agents like psyllium husk can assist absorb excess water in the digestive tract and encourage firmer stools, while antidiarrheal drugs like loperamide can help slow down colon transit time and lessen urgency. Before beginning any new supplement or pharmaceutical regimen, it is imperative to speak with a healthcare provider, as they can offer tailored advice based on each person's needs and medical background.

All things considered, managing constipation after ileoanal pouch surgery necessitates a multimodal strategy that includes dietary changes, lifestyle improvements, and, if required, medicinal measures. As they adjust to the changes in their digestive systems, people can effectively control their symptoms and enhance their general quality of life by putting these ideas into practice.

CHAPTER 5
RECIPES AND FOOD SELECTIONS

An appropriate diet is essential for the healing process and long-term health of patients after ileoanal pouch surgery. During the ileoanal pouch operation, a small intestine pouch is created to hold feces after the colon and rectum are removed owing to disorders like familial adenomatous polyposis or ulcerative colitis. For patients to recuperate, avoid complications, and have the best possible outcome, post-surgery nutrition is crucial. We will discuss the significance of dietary decisions and recipes designed to assist patients having ileoanal pouch surgery in this extensive guide.

Gentle and Simple Recipes

Following ileoanal pouch surgery, individuals frequently have short-term digestive difficulties while their bodies get used to the altered bowel function.

To reduce discomfort and promote optimal nutrient absorption, it is imperative to include soft, easily digested meals in the post-surgery diet. Patients recovering from surgery can easily accept soft foods, which are easy on the digestive system and include boiled vegetables, mashed potatoes, rice, muesli, and tender meats or fish.

Incorporating soluble fiber-rich foods like cooked carrots, applesauce, and bananas can also help control bowel movements and stave against constipation without placing undue strain on the recently formed pouch. Easy-to-digest proteins, such as eggs, tofu, and cooked poultry, can also aid in tissue repair and the body's healing process. Patients can make sure that their nutritional demands are satisfied while minimizing gastrointestinal discomfort throughout the recovery phase by concentrating on soft and easy-to-digest dishes.

While it's crucial to include soft, easily digested meals in your post-surgery diet, it's also critical to stay away from items that could make your symptoms worse or lead to complications.

Foods that can be difficult for people with an ileoanal pouch to digest include fresh fruits and vegetables, seeds, nuts, and tough pieces of meat.

These foods can also raise the risk of pouchitis or bowel blockages. As a result, it's advised that patients stay away from certain meals when they're first recovering and then return them to their diet as tolerated. Patients can choose easier-to-digest prepared or canned fruits and vegetables in place of raw ones. Comparably, substituting lean, tender meat pieces or substitutes like fish or tofu for rough cuts might help avoid stomach pain while still offering vital nutrients.

Patients should also steer clear of diets heavy in processed components, artificial sweeteners, and added sugars as they might aggravate inflammation and compromise gut health. Patients can reduce the risk of problems and optimize their post-surgery diet by identifying and avoiding trigger foods.

Delicious and Nutritious Dinner Ideas

Long-term adherence to a post-surgery nutrition plan is contingent upon the maintenance of a delicious and diverse diet. Patients can still enjoy a variety of tasty and healthy meals that support healing and general well-being, even though the emphasis is on soft and simple-to-digest cuisine. Herbs, spices, and sauces such as ginger, turmeric, garlic, and lemon juice can enhance the taste and texture of food without overpowering the stomach. Trying out various cooking techniques, including boiling, steaming, or baking, can also improve the flavor and texture of food while making sure it stays easy on the stomach. Patients can have scrambled eggs with spinach and feta cheese or muesli with mashed banana and cinnamon for breakfast. Lunch and dinner options that encourage healing and increase satiety include vegetable soup with shredded chicken, quinoa salad with roasted vegetables, and baked salmon with mashed sweet potatoes. After ileoanal pouch surgery, patients can support their long-term nutritional objectives and maintain a positive relationship with food by prioritizing wholesome and enjoyable meal options.

selecting foods and dishes that promote healing and long-term wellness is crucial when navigating the post-surgical diet following ileoanal pouch surgery. Patients can maximize their nutrition and reduce the risk of problems while supporting healing and overall well-being by including soft and easy-to-digest foods, avoiding trigger foods, and embracing tasty and nourishing meal ideas. Having close collaboration with trained dietitians and healthcare professionals can offer extra direction and assistance in creating a customized nutrition plan that suits each person's requirements and preferences. Following ileoanal pouch surgery, patients can experience optimal results and a great quality of life with appropriate nutrition and dietary management.

CHAPTER 6
SPECIAL DIETARY CONSIDERATIONS

For patients having ileoanal pouch surgery, certain food guidelines are crucial for promoting the best possible healing and long-term health. Individualized nutrition planning is essential in this context, since patients may have particular dietary needs or limits depending on their medical background, personal preferences, and stage of recuperation following surgery.

A customized strategy is necessary to tailor nutrition for individual needs, taking into consideration things like food allergies, intolerances, digestive problems, and nutritional deficits. For instance, some patients might need to stay away from items that make their gastrointestinal problems worse, while others might need more nutrients to help with tissue repair and wound healing. People can develop a customized nutrition plan that fits their needs and encourages the best possible health results by speaking with a registered dietitian or nutritionist.

For those having ileoanal pouch surgery, gluten-free and dairy-free choices are frequently advised because these dietary changes can help lessen inflammation and alleviate stomach issues.

Wheat, barley, and rye include gluten, which some people find difficult to digest and which can cause gastrointestinal distress or aggravate pre-existing inflammation in the digestive tract. Likewise, individuals who are lactose intolerant or have sensitivities to dairy proteins may experience digestive problems after consuming lactose-containing dairy products. People can help maintain the health of their digestive systems and reduce pain while recovering by choosing plant-based milk, dairy-free cheese, and gluten-free and dairy-free grains.

For those having ileoanal pouch surgery, vegetarian and vegan modifications are also crucial to take into account. This is especially true for those who adhere to plant-based diets for moral, environmental, or health reasons. A diet rich in minerals and antioxidants that promote healing and general well-being can be found in vegetarian and vegan diets.

But it's crucial to make sure these diets are well-balanced and full of different plant-based protein sources, such as whole grains, beans, lentils, tofu, and tempeh. Consuming an abundance of fruits, vegetables, and leafy greens can also help people achieve their micronutrient requirements and encourage the best possible recovery following surgery. Making a balanced meal plan that satisfies one's dietary preferences and health objectives might be made easier by working with a dietitian or nutritionist who specializes in vegetarian and vegan nutrition.

patients having ileoanal pouch surgery require specific dietary considerations, such as individualized nutrition plans, dairy- and gluten-free alternatives, and vegetarian and vegan modifications. By tailoring diet regimens to each person's requirements and tastes, people can minimise gastrointestinal distress, aid in the healing process, and advance long-term wellness.

A competent healthcare provider, such as a certified dietitian or nutritionist, can offer invaluable advice and assistance in managing dietary adjustments and maximizing nutrient intake for the best possible health results.

CHAPTER 7
SUPPLEMENTS AND VITAMINS

Understanding the function of vitamins and supplements in the context of ileoanal pouch surgery nutrition is essential for guaranteeing the best possible health and well-being following surgery.

To promote healing, avoid problems, and preserve general health, the surgical procedure—which entails creating an internal reservoir from the small intestine to replace the resected colon and rectum—requires close attention to nutritional intake.

In this extensive guide, we discuss the importance of vitamins and supplements, list suggested nutrients, and offer tips on how to successfully include them in your diet after surgery.

After ileoanal pouch surgery, patients frequently have altered digestive systems and reduced capacity to absorb nutrients.

The efficiency with which the body absorbs vital vitamins and minerals from food can be affected by surgical modifications made to the gastrointestinal system. Consequently, there is an increased requirement for supplements to close any possible nutritional gaps and support optimum health.

It's important to understand your individual supplement needs, which usually entails speaking with doctors, dietitians, and gastroenterologists among other healthcare specialists. The extent of surgery, dietary habits, past medical history, and present health state are all important considerations for creating customized supplement regimens. Furthermore, understanding the significance of supplement quality, purity, and bioavailability guarantees that you get the most out of these dietary additions.

Suggested Minerals and Vitamins

Including a wide range of vitamins and minerals in your diet after surgery is crucial for maintaining many physiological processes and enhancing general health. Important nutrients that are frequently advised after ileoanal pouch surgery consist of, but are not restricted to:

1.Vitamin B12: Due to possible malabsorption problems during surgery, vitamin B12 supplementation may be necessary. Vitamin B12 is essential for brain function and the production of red blood cells.

2. Iron: Enough iron consumption is essential for boosting the body's ability to carry oxygen throughout its tissues and preventing anemia. Supplemental iron may be necessary for those with ileoanal pouches to make up for their reduced ability to absorb iron.

3. Calcium and Vitamin D: Supplementing with calcium and vitamin D may be important to support bone health and muscle function, particularly if dairy intake is restricted or malabsorption problems occur.

4. Probiotics: Good bacteria are essential for preserving gut health and facilitating digestion. Probiotic pills may help alleviate symptoms like bloating and diarrhea by restoring the microbial balance in the gastrointestinal system.

5. The anti-inflammatory qualities of omega-3 fatty acids help to lower inflammation and improve cardiovascular health. For those suffering from pouch-related inflammation or inflammatory bowel disease (IBD), supplementing with fish oil or algae-based sources may be helpful.

How to Include Supplements in Your Diet

Including supplements in your diet after surgery calls for careful preparation and following medical advice.

To create a customized regimen that meets your unique needs, start by talking with your healthcare provider about your specific supplement needs.

As you add new items to your daily routine, think about things like dosage, time, and possible interactions with other supplements or prescriptions.

Select premium supplements from reliable producers to guarantee efficacy, safety, and purity. Moreover, make an effort to consume supplements consistently by following the suggested quantities and frequency as directed by medical professionals. Optimizing your nutrient status and promoting long-term wellness requires that you keep an eye on how you respond to supplements and modify your routine as necessary in response to regular assessments and input from your healthcare team.

following ileoanal pouch surgery, navigating the world of vitamins and supplements calls for a thorough assessment of each patient's unique needs, expert advice, and adherence to recommended supplementing techniques. Through comprehension of supplement needs, setting important nutrients as top priorities, and carefully incorporating supplements into your diet, you can facilitate recovery, improve nutritional status, and foster long-term health and well-being after surgery.

CHAPTER 8
WELL-BEING LIFESTYLE TIPS

A person's lifestyle is very important for their recovery after surgery, especially if they have ileoanal pouch surgery. Healthy habits can greatly improve general well-being, facilitate the healing process, and support long-term health when incorporated into everyday routines. This section will include a variety of lifestyle advice, including suggestions for physical activity and exercise, ways to handle stress, and ways to improve the quality of your sleep.

Exercise and Guidelines for Physical Activity

Regular physical activity and exercise are crucial for patients healing after ileoanal pouch surgery. Before beginning any fitness program, it is crucial to start slowly and speak with medical professionals. First, simple exercises like walking or light stretching can aid in promoting healing, enhancing circulation, and averting problems like blood clots. Swimming, cycling, or low-impact aerobics are examples of gradually introducing increasingly strenuous activities as recuperation advances and the person's strength grows.

Exercises for strengthening the core muscles through resistance training can also be helpful since they support the surgery site and increase abdominal strength. However, it's important to stay away from exercises that strain or apply excessive pressure to the abdominal region, particularly in the early phases after rehabilitation. Engaging with a licensed trainer or physical therapist can offer individualized advice and guarantee that workouts are secure and suitable for each person's requirements.

When it comes to exercise after surgery, consistency is essential. Regular exercise regimens that gradually increase in time and intensity can help improve mood, increase physical fitness, and improve general well-being. Sustaining an appropriate diet and hydration is also essential for promoting post-exercise recovery and maximizing results.

Techniques for Stress Management

For those recuperating from ileoanal pouch surgery, stress management is crucial because stress can impair recovery and general health. Using stress-reduction strategies can ease tension, encourage relaxation, and enhance mental health. Stress reduction and mental calmness can be achieved by practices including gradual muscle relaxation, yoga, meditation, and deep breathing exercises.

Finding and addressing sources of stress in daily life—whether they have to do with relationships, the workplace, or health issues—is also crucial. People who practice mindfulness and maintain present-moment awareness are better able to manage stress and develop inner calm. In addition, partaking in joyful and fulfilling pursuits like hobbies, quality time with loved ones, or outdoor activities can aid in stress relief and enhance general well-being.

Getting help from loved ones, friends, or support groups can also help reduce stress during recovery. Talking to people who understand your experiences, worries, and feelings can help you feel validated, inspired, and able to offer helpful guidance. Additionally, those who are under a lot of stress or are having trouble overcoming the obstacles of rehabilitation may find that professional counseling or therapy is beneficial.

Improving the Quality of Your Sleep

For general health and well-being, especially in the post-ileoanal pouch surgery healing phase, getting enough sleep is crucial. On the other hand, a lot of people could have trouble sleeping because of surgical pain, discomfort, or anxiety.

Putting techniques to increase sleep quality into practice can help with mood, healing, and general recovery.

Better sleep patterns can be encouraged by establishing a regular sleep schedule and bedtime ritual, which can assist control the body's internal clock. This entails having a consistent bedtime and wake-up time every day in addition to doing peaceful things like reading, having a warm bath, or practicing relaxation techniques in the evening.

Encouraging peaceful sleep also requires creating a cozy sleeping environment. Making sure the bedroom is peaceful, dark, and at a suitable temperature is part of this. Purchasing pillows and a supportive mattress can also aid in reducing pain and encouraging improved sleeping posture.

Reducing your intake of stimulants like nicotine, caffeine, and electronics before bed will help you unwind and get better sleep. Sleep patterns can also be avoided by reducing alcohol intake and avoiding big meals or snacks right before bed.

It's crucial to speak with medical professionals if sleep difficulties continue after trying these remedies to rule out any underlying medical conditions or pharmaceutical side effects that might be causing the issue. They can offer direction and suggestions for dealing with sleep problems and encouraging improved general sleep hygiene.

adopting wellness-promoting lifestyle practices is crucial for patients recuperating after ileoanal pouch surgery. People can facilitate the healing process, advance long-term health, and enhance general well-being by making exercise and physical activity a priority, putting stress management strategies into practice, and improving the quality of their sleep. Seeking advice and recommendations from healthcare specialists that are specific to each person's requirements and situation is crucial.

CHAPTER 9
LONG-TERM NUTRITION MAINTENANCE

Maintaining Nutritious Health After Rehabilitation:

Maintaining ideal nutritional health becomes crucial for long-term well-being following ileoanal pouch surgery. This surgery includes removing the colon and creating an internal pouch from the small intestine to replace its function. It is frequently used to treat illnesses like ulcerative colitis or familial adenomatous polyposis.

Although the procedure relieves crippling symptoms, it also alters the way the digestive system functions, requiring close attention to diet to maintain health.

Patients need to concentrate on maintaining an appropriate diet after surgery to aid in healing, avert problems, and enhance general health. This means following a nutritionally balanced diet that satisfies each person's unique demands while taking into account any dietary recommendations made by medical professionals.

Maintaining appropriate food intake becomes crucial for maximizing immune system performance, digestive function, and general quality of life while the body adapts to surgical changes.

Modest Dietary Changes Over Time:

The path to the best post-surgery diet is a dynamic one that calls for little changes made over time rather than a static one. Patients may need to adhere to a temporarily limited diet in the early postoperative phases to give the pouch time to recover and adjust to its new role.

This could entail eating meals that are simple to digest, avoiding trigger foods that might make symptoms worse, and reintroducing solid foods gradually as tolerated.

Patients can collaborate with healthcare providers, such as registered dietitians or nutritionists, to gradually increase their food choices while making sure they are getting enough nutrients while their bodies heal and adjust to the pouch.

This procedure is keeping an eye on each person's tolerance to various meals, figuring out any dietary triggers or intolerances, and adjusting the diet as necessary. Patients can optimize their nutritional intake while minimizing the risk of stomach pain or consequences by implementing individualized, progressive dietary adjustments.

Keeping an eye on and handling any complications: Ileoanal pouch surgery has the potential to cause complications that could affect nutritional health, but it can also greatly enhance quality of life for people with specific gastrointestinal issues. Pouchitis, or inflammation of the internal pouch, is a common consequence that can result in symptoms like diarrhea, abdominal pain, and poor nutrition absorption.

Additionally, due to changes in digestive function following surgery, patients may encounter problems like dehydration, electrolyte imbalances, or vitamin shortages.

Patients must have regular monitoring by medical professionals, including follow-up visits with surgeons, gastroenterologists, and dietitians, to minimize these consequences and preserve optimal nutritional health. Monitoring may include measuring symptoms, measuring nutritional levels in the blood, and measuring pouch function via imaging scans. To treat difficulties and advance long-term wellness, healthcare professionals might suggest suitable therapies, such as dietary changes, supplementation, or medication, based on the findings.

a comprehensive strategy that takes into account the particular dietary requirements and difficulties related to ileoanal pouch surgery is necessary to achieve and maintain good nutritional health after the surgical treatment. Patients can assist in healing, prevent nutritional deficits, and promote long-term wellness by focusing on maintaining nutritional health beyond the recovery period, gradually adjusting their diet over time, and monitoring and managing any issues. Working together with medical specialists is crucial to overcoming the challenges of post-surgery nutrition and providing each patient with the individualized care and support they need to lead a healthy and full life.

CONCLUSION

Taking a holistic approach to nutrition and wellbeing is necessary to successfully navigate the post-surgery recovery process. From comprehending the nuances of ileoanal pouch surgery to adopting a customized diet after surgery, this book has offered priceless information and tools to those starting this recuperation process.

We've covered the critical role that nutrition plays in promoting the best possible recovery throughout the chapters, stressing the significance of pre-operative planning and post-surgery nutritional progression. We've talked about how to effectively manage digestive issues, prepare nutritious, well-balanced meals, and easily handle unique dietary needs.

Through the integration of professional advice, therapeutic recipes, and meal planning, patients can set out on a journey toward sustained wellbeing following surgery. Every facet of nutrition, from minimizing dietary discomfort to maximizing micronutrient intake, has been thoroughly thought out to aid in healing and advance general health.

Moreover, this book covers lifestyle variables that are critical for overall health in addition to nutritional advice.

Through advice for exercise and stress management strategies, people are empowered to improve their quality of life and build resilience while they pursue recovery.

By adhering to the guidelines provided in this extensive manual, we not only give priority to the immediate recovery following surgery, but we also provide the groundwork for long-term nutritional health. Through careful observation and management of possible side effects and incremental dietary modifications over time, people can develop a robust and flourishing lifestyle that lasts well beyond recovery.

Essentially, this manual acts as a beacon of hope and direction, giving people the information and resources, they need to confidently and resiliently negotiate the challenges of post-surgery eating.

By dedicating themselves to self-care, holistic wellness, and proper nutrition, people can welcome a future full of energy and well-being.